# The Lyons Report
# 2020

## by Theresa Lyons MS, MS, PhD

Dr. Theresa Lyons

The Lyons Report

ISBN 978-1-7343582-0-9

Library of Congress Control Number: 2020901980

# Contents

# **Dedication**

This book is dedicated to:

All those with autism who want to feel better. You can.

All the parents who know their child understands everything.
You're right. They do.

All the healthcare practitioners who do their best to help.
Thank you.

To my Uncle Joe, whose inspiration lives on.

.

# **Introduction**

## DISCLOSURE

By reading this book, I hereby understand and agree that The
Lyons Report and Navigating AWEtism is not endorsing any of
these practitioners. All medical advice, treatment, and/or products
and services given by those listed in The Lyons Report will be taken
by me utilizing my own discretion after a thorough investigation
and assessment as to whether that practitioner is suitable and
competent to assist me with my or my child's health needs. I do
not and will not hold Navigating AWEtism or Dr. Theresa Lyons
responsible in any way for the background, education, licensure,
scope of practice, claims history, or clinical expertise of any
practitioner I may contact as a result of using this guidebook.
Should I experience an unsatisfactory outcome of care with
anyone named in this report, I will not hold Navigating AWEtism
or Dr. Theresa Lyons responsible for that outcome.

The Lyons Report has no means of continually monitoring these
listed practitioners and their relative training or licensure status
or claims history, or if their style or method of practice is suitable
for me or my child. Selecting a practitioner from The Lyons Report
is not a substitute for a thorough investigation of my chosen
clinician's professional degree and training, clinical experience,
scope of practice, insurance reimbursement options, and other
factors that may weigh in my decision of who to work with.
The Lyons Report does not verify or investigate the education
or credentials of the people listed.  This guide book does not

advise me about any particular clinician's expertise or scope of practice.  The Lyons Report does not provide compensated recommendations.

Theresa Lyons MS, MS, PhD

Dear Reader,

*Welcome!*

If you're holding this book in your hands (or reading it on your e-reader), then congratulations. You've just taken an important step toward developing an effective healing plan for your child with autism.

I want you to know that there *is* hope.

You have more control than you may realize as you strive to help your child.

Wherever you are on the journey right now, you've undoubtedly heard of Functional Medicine. Maybe you've heard from other parents about how it's helping their children, or from a practitioner. If you have, you've also likely heard how effective it can be in uncovering and healing the causes of some of your child's symptoms. But when it comes to finding a provider who knows what he or she is doing (and determining whether he or she is a good match for your child), you may feel a bit overwhelmed.

Take a deep breath and keep reading—you're in good hands now!

I'd like to tell you a little bit about my own story, so you know how I'm qualified to guide you on your journey with autism—and

*why it's my personal mission to provide you with a sense of hope
along with the quality information I'm sharing.*

I'm Dr. Theresa Lyons, the Professor of Healing Autism, and the
parent of a daughter who has made great strides toward healing
from autism.

A world-renowned autism doctor diagnosed my daughter with
severe autism when she was three and-a-half; now, six years later,
she's a different child; one who laughs, loves going on adventures,
and is fierce about learning.

My own journey has led me to where I am now: on a mission to
*help other parents find (or rediscover) the joy in parenting as they
do the work to heal their children.*

*Parent to parent, I want to inspire you with what's possible.*

My clients—the parents of children with autism—have seen
significant changes in the health and well-being of their children.

What could this healing look like for you, as a parent? I recently
heard from one of my clients—a husband-and-wife team—that
they actually sat down and drank coffee together as a couple.
(Since you're here, reading this right now, I know I don't have to
tell you how big of a deal that is!) For years, their eight-year-old
son had been a constant source of worry. He was destructive, so
they had to constantly be within arm's reach.

I worked with the parents on a new diet, making sure they felt supported. I helped them find a new Functional Medicine doctor who removed unnecessary medications and supplements. We focused on optimizing the son's body chemistry, and the subtle changes we made created significant improvements in his behavior within three months.

In fact, on one recent Sunday morning, after he'd been on the adjusted diet and off some of those medications and supplements for a little while, he went outside and played with his sister and a friend—something that had rarely, if ever, happened. They were playing so nicely together! And for the first time in as long as they could remember, the boy's parents wondered what they'd do with their free time. The husband rushed into the house to make them a cup of coffee, and as they sat together, they looked at each other and laughed. The husband said to his wife, "Is *this* what parenting is like?"

In this case, as in every case, building a healthcare team (the Functional Medicine practitioner and me) was important, because before the parents began their work with me, they felt like no one believed their son could improve. But I believed he could … and with the parents' efforts to make changes and optimize his body chemistry, he did!

This isn't an isolated account of success, either. I'm honored to have helped many parents have wonderful family experiences. Like my client who told me how her family—all five of them!—went on a Disney cruise and had a blast! It was so great to hear about how they were able to just have fun. Their child with autism slept through the night, handled transitions well, enjoyed the cruise activities, and even ate new food. Plus, everybody now has such great memories!

**When you do the work to heal your child, your parenting experience changes, dramatically; you're able to step out of the caretaker role and just enjoy parenting your child.**

# MY STORY

My intuition first started telling me something was "off" when my daughter was about nine months old. Parenting was *really* hard. The bond we had established started to vanish. She didn't look at me when I walked into a room. She didn't smile at me, greet me, or say goodbye. It was hard for me to connect with her. And I felt very, very isolated.

Her doctors wanted to be very thorough. Although they were thinking autism was a possibility, they wanted to make sure they considered and eliminated anything else. We spent quite a bit of time doing testing and evaluations during this "investigative stage."

When my daughter was a toddler, she had some words, and then lost them. She wasn't talking very much at all. When I talked to her regular pediatrician about it during her wellness checks, she said I needed to read to my daughter more, and the doctor asked how much time I spent away from my daughter.

I felt angry and guilty … angry that the doctor was insinuating my daughter wasn't thriving because of something I was neglecting, and guilty because, at the time, I was a perfectionist, and I thought I might not be doing the best possible job of parenting.

I tried all the things the pediatrician recommended, like saying, "banana" when I fed her a banana, reading her more "child-friendly" books (instead of the science journals we'd both loved reading together), and taking her to more activities where she had a chance to socialize with other children.

Even though I thought I was doing everything "right," my daughter wasn't speaking, writing, or smiling. She had meltdowns, noise sensitivity, light sensitivity, seizures, and aggressive behavior. She didn't feel pain, and couldn't sit still. She was withdrawn, and *everything* felt difficult.

I felt like a failure.

Eventually, when my daughter was about three and-a-half, a specialist diagnosed my daughter with severe autism.

I remember instantly mourning the loss of her childhood. I felt so sorry for her that she'd never have a typical life—no friends, no real schooling, no prom. I felt sorry for myself, too! I wondered what her diagnosis meant for me, how I'd live through it.

It seemed unfair to both of us.

Of course, I longed to connect with her. I wanted, more than anything, to share special moments with her, to see her laugh and enjoy life. All parents have fantasies about what they'll do with their children. Runners dream of running as a family. Outdoor enthusiasts dream of hiking with their kids, pointing out different flora and fauna, being surprised by their child's level of understanding and curiosity. Personally, I loved tea parties as a child, so I imagined playing dress-up with my daughter and having fancy tea parties and, when she got older, spa days.

We *all* want to know we provided a great childhood for our children. Right?

Before I did anything to help her, though, I wanted to know if she *wanted* my help.

So, one day, I gave her a piece of paper and some finger paints while she was sitting in her highchair. I said to her, "If this is who you are, I can love you this way. But if you want me to help you, then you've got to give me some signs, so I know I do what you want."

She took her hands and moved them around and made this big heart on the paper. She had never made anything artistic before, so to me, this heart was an absolute clear sign that she wanted help.

To me, she was saying she wanted something *different*. She wanted to feel better. She wanted me to take action and help her.

That was my North Star.

From that moment forward, I knew nothing would stand in my way of discovering what autism is, on a scientific level. I knew nothing would stand in my way of helping her heal.

# MY FIRST STEPS

Before I was ever a parent, I was a scientist. I earned my Ph.D. in chemistry from Yale University, and worked for years in the U.S. healthcare industry as a researcher and a healthcare strategist. I knew science and I knew the healthcare system; this gave me comfort in knowing how to start helping my daughter.

And I got right to work.

Whenever I'm facing a difficult problem, the most important thing for me is to come up to speed on information.

I decided to leverage my professional skills as a scientist and a researcher to help my daughter. I read all the scientific literature I could get my hands on—papers and studies the public didn't have access to. Then I used my medical strategy skills to build a team of world-renowned specialists to help my daughter. (This is huge—I knew I'd be able to ask questions most people wouldn't get answers to for 30 years.)

At the time, the word "healing," wasn't in my vocabulary as a potential end result for my daughter. I just knew I wanted her to get better. But once I started understanding the science behind all her symptoms—digestive issues, pain, and other aspects—the word "healing" became accurate.

You see, it wasn't about trying to change her or "stamp out" her autism … it was about improving her quality of life.

My goal became thinking about her autism in a compassionate way—and helping her to heal, to gain an "optimal outcome."

Next, I began to seek out other parents who had healed their children from autism. I began to hear a quiet whisper … *"Your child doesn't have to be autistic her whole life."*

In talking with these parents, I got to sense their results—feel, hear, taste, touch, and smell. Their stories gave me anecdotal evidence that healing was possible. That evidence, combined with what the research showed was possible, gave me the hope I needed to begin taking even bigger steps to heal my daughter.

Plus, having supportive people around me made all the difference. I finally felt like I wasn't the only one who saw my daughter's potential and who truly believed she could heal; these people became her advocates *and* mine.

And over time, as I implemented everything I learned into my daughter's care (including Functional Medicine, a vital part of healing autism, which I get into more detail about below), she *did* begin to heal. She became more functional, more interactive, more expressive. As she improved, we celebrated her successes (which is one element of the Autism Healing Matrix)—and we both *enjoyed* it! For so long, I hadn't smiled or laughed. But now, we were enjoying life again, and it was so amazing.

I finally felt like a parent again, rather than like a caretaker! My entire life changed.

The truth is, we were all inspired. The doctors I worked with encouraged me to teach what I'd learned to other parents. And while that's what I set out to do, initially, I soon found that in addition to teaching, *supporting* parents was really important, too.

Now, I'm so happy to say that through information and inspiration, I'm helping parents all over the world to help their children heal! And I can help you, too.

As I've worked and spoken with more and more parents of children who have an autism diagnosis, I've realized that many parents are hearing about Functional Medicine. They have a high-level understanding of what it is, but they want to know more … and they want to know how to choose a practitioner who will be a good match for their child.

That's why I decided to write this book: to give you a little more information about Functional Medicine, and to offer you a list of

Functional Medicine practitioners by state *who want to work with those with autism.*

An important note: Each of the doctors in this book is an MD. I looked at their training in either Functional Medicine or Integrative Medicine to ensure they care for and optimize the functioning of the child's entire body (not just the gut or brain or liver, but the whole body, since everything is connected).

Either my clients have used these doctors themselves (which is the case with many of the doctors in this book, so I have first-hand knowledge of how they practice), or I've spoken with them personally to ask how they address working with a child with autism. Some of them have been healing children with autism for over 40 years, and some are just beginning; however, each and every one of them believes that so much more is possible for children with autism. This is the kind of expert you want on your child's healthcare team … someone who believes in your child's future. And that's why I'd love to connect you with him or her!

A doctor can't buy his or her way onto this list; in fact, none of the doctors knew they were included on this list until I called and told them (this is important, because many "Top Doctor" lists are just marketing ploys doctors can pay to be featured on).

Finally, I want you to know that I would take my own daughter to any of the doctors in this book.

When I first learned about Functional Medicine, I loved what I heard. The science is solid, and it is how physicians used to practice medicine: by investigating and treating the root cause. It's about investing time, energy, and money into the future.

However, as I started to expand my daughter's healthcare team, I evaluated each potential team member to determine whether he or she was a good fit. I scoffed at any doctor who didn't take insurance. I (erroneously) assumed these doctors were in medicine just to make money. I thought insurance companies knew what was best for my daughter (I later realized that insurance companies know how to make a profit, but they don't really have my daughter's best interests in mind).

Because of my erroneous beliefs, I lost precious time as I began the journey of helping my daughter to heal.

In my research, I interviewed several parents who used Functional Medicine to help their children. I finally decided to take my daughter to a Functional Medicine practitioner and spent about a year interviewing several before finally choosing one. The first two appointments cost $1200—before any testing or treatments—which seemed like a huge investment. In many ways, I kept worrying that I'd waste money if nothing changed. Even though I knew guarantees aren't possible in the medical world, I wished for one!

*It was so worth it.* Working with a knowledgeable Functional Medicine practitioner made *all* the difference.

I wish I'd had someone to explain all of this to me early on, so that my daughter's health could have improved even faster.

And that's another reason I'm writing this book: to save you and your child that time.

It *is* that important.

Now, let's talk more about Functional Medicine.

# WHAT IS FUNCTIONAL MEDICINE?

According to The Institute for Functional Medicine, "Functional Medicine determines how and why illness occurs and restores health by addressing the root causes of disease for each individual. It is a systems biology-based approach to medicine that focuses on identifying and addressing the root cause of disease. Each symptom or differential diagnosis may be one of many contributing to a person's illness."

A diagnosis can be the result of more than one cause. The precise manifestation of each cause depends on the individual's genes, environment, and lifestyle, and only treatments that address the right cause and optimize all three components will have lasting benefit beyond symptom suppression.

The Functional Medicine Model evolved from the insights and perspectives of a small group of thought leaders who realized the importance of an individualized approach to disease causes.

They found ways to apply these new advances to use low-risk interventions that modify molecular and cellular systems to reverse drivers of disease.

In many cases, the results were wonderful: patients who had previously received unsuccessful treatments often experienced dramatic improvements.

# HOW IS FUNCTIONAL MEDICINE DIFFERENT FROM CONVENTIONAL MEDICINE?

Functional Medicine and Conventional Medicine each play an important role in the healing process, and it's best to use both approaches during this journey.

In many ways, Functional Medicine and Conventional Medicine are similar. Licensed medical professionals practice both, both are evidence-based and scientific, and both use diagnostic testing to determine underlying causes of symptoms.

Often, Conventional Medicine does a great job of addressing acute and urgent medical conditions like broken bones, acute illnesses (colds, sinus infections, strep throat, etc.), and other trauma. Skilled doctors and physicians in the Conventional Medicine field may focus on using prescription medications or surgery to help their patients.

**On the other hand, Functional Medicine operates on the belief that the body has an innate ability to heal itself,** and is often used to treat chronic or ongoing symptoms, like gastrointestinal issues, fatigue, recurring pains, and more. Rather than simply treating the symptoms, though, Functional Medicine addresses the underlying causes of disease, using a systems-oriented approach to identify and begin correcting imbalances in the body that lead to the symptoms.

# WHY TREAT WITH FUNCTIONAL MEDICINE?

So many of the parents I talk with report that their child's regular blood tests came back "normal," and that the doctors tell them the child has autism and is "otherwise healthy."

But the parents know something isn't right. They know their child isn't well.

Autism is *so* complex, and frequently, it affects the body as a whole. Unless they're specially trained in how the body's systems relate to and affect one another, many doctors don't know exactly what to look for.

Because Functional Medicine looks at the body as a whole system rather than a collection of organs, it's a great way to approach and treat autism. It goes beyond routine, using advanced diagnostic testing to discern how a person's body is functioning as a system. So rather than simple blood tests, a Functional Medicine doctor would likely test things like stool and urine, look for environmental toxins, nutrient deficiencies and inflammation, and consider genetics.

When I explain Functional Medicine testing results to parents, I paint a picture of how their child's body is operating, and how specific test results relate to some "autism behaviors."

For example, the gut microbiota produces certain molecules that can correlate to some autism behaviors. Functional Medicine testing can reveal what those molecules are, so the doctor can then create an individual treatment plan to address that specific issue. This is how Functional Medicine takes an individual systems approach to healing.

Autism is a spectrum, as you probably know. This means that some people who have autism symptoms may be "low-functioning," and need more intervention and assistance. Their autism-related behaviors might be more obvious and severe, and they may need to be enrolled in special education programs at school or need assistance as adults. Other people with autism symptoms may be "high-functioning." They may be placed in mainstream classrooms, and their autism-related behaviors may not be as pronounced or obvious.

An autism diagnosis is based on observation—that's why many people think of "autism" as a behavior.

But a deeper scientific understanding of the autism spectrum reveals that there's much more to this diagnosis than behavior.

Consider that on one hand; about nine percent of people diagnosed with autism eventually heal completely. They show no signs or symptoms of autism. On the other hand, literature and research shows that the life expectancy of people with autism is drastically reduced. In the U.S., for example, a 2017 analysis showed that people with autism who died between 1999 and 2014 had a mean age of 36 at the time of death, while the general population's mean age at death is twice that: 72.

What does this mean?

It means that for people who have autism, there is so much more than behavior that will affect quality of life.

Swedish researchers looking at life expectancy found that people with low-functioning autism most often died from seizures, while people with high-functioning autism most often died from suicide. The bottom line is that autism affects quality of life and length of life, for myriad different reasons.

That's why it's so important to seek a varied set of resources—including top-notch Conventional and Functional Medicine practitioners—as you work to help your child heal.

# THE POWER IN PARTNERSHIPS

Helping your child heal from autism is about maximizing all the resources available.

Earlier, I mentioned my Autism Healing Matrix, which outlines the different areas, or components—you must address on the healing journey, including:

1. Diet.

2. Healthcare team.

3. Supportive environment.

4. Supplements.

5. Educational approaches.

6. Probiotics.

7. Celebrate success.

All of these components work synergistically.

Autism and the healing process are much like an orchestra—many components coming together to create a result … a wonderful blend of sounds and sights that make you feel truly alive and grateful.

Imagine an orchestral performance. Each component—the velvet seating, the cool, dark theater, the building's high ceilings, acoustics, and majestic architecture, the different sounds created by the strings, woodwinds, brass, and percussion, the conductor—

works in synergy with the others to create a complete experience for each audience member.

Now, close your eyes and imagine someone hitting "play" on Louis Armstrong's "What a Wonderful World." Six instruments— the violin, drum, flute, double bass, trumpet, and harpsichord— combine with the deepness of Louis' voice, and you feel like you're floating on a cloud … *"I see trees of green …"*

That's the kind of synergy you leverage with the Autism Healing Matrix! And when all of its components come together in a crescendo, you get results. Like the song says, *"What a wonderful world!"*

As you can see, healthcare team is just one of the Matrix's components. Creating a team is such an elegant, necessary move on the healing journey (just like all the other components are, too).

Trying to do this all on your own will literally exhaust you to the point of a major health crisis as you spend all your time in caregiver mode (rather than a parent mode). You cannot heal autism all on your own (and if you think that it's your sole responsibility, it becomes burdensome, and it's hard to do it in a compassionate way).

Creating a team gives you access to professionals who can see every component of your child and how all the elements come together, from diet to probiotics to supplements to behaviors to emotional support.

While all the members of the team are equally important, the focus of this book is to help you find a Functional Medicine practitioner you can trust to help you heal your child.

That being said, I recommend that your healthcare team include practitioners from both Conventional Medicine and Functional Medicine. Both types of medicine play an important role in helping your child heal from autism.

As I mentioned earlier, Conventional Medicine is great for providing immediate care for common issues and helping to identify underlying medical problems.

Meanwhile, Functional Medicine strives to get to the very root of what's causing your child's symptoms, and to take a personalized approach to healing those root causes.

Together, Conventional Medicine and Functional Medicine have the power to improve your child's quality of life.

That's why Functional and Conventional Medicine complement each other so well, and why I recommend including doctors from both camps in your child's healing plan. You want an expert in each of the many realms of healing autism, so you can get the best information and make the best decisions.

# A NOTE ABOUT INSURANCE

As I mentioned earlier, I initially balked at pursuing Functional Medicine practitioners for my daughter's care, because not many of them accepted insurance. If you feel this way, too, I completely understand. If you've been on this autism healing journey for any length of time, you've probably invested lots of money in co-pays, supplements, different therapies, and other tools to help your child.

Spending even more on a visit to a doctor who doesn't take insurance can feel like such a stretch!

But I want to reiterate that the advice you'll receive from such a practitioner is worth the investment, and will likely save you money in the long run as you begin to see improvements in your child's symptoms.

Think of it this way: one of my clients recently called me to tell me her son said "thank you" to her—unprompted!—for the very first time. While this might seem insignificant to some, you and I know how important it really is! This spontaneous "thank you" showed what a kind and loving son she was raising and made her believe that her son is smart and learning. And these are the kinds of things that I see happening all the time in my work that make investments in your child's care trivial and irrelevant.

Plus, a greater number of Functional Medicine practitioners are starting to take insurance. Specifically, the Cleveland Clinic's

Center for Functional Medicine bills insurance and is leading the way in changing some aspects of healthcare.

# HOW TO USE THE INFORMATION IN THIS BOOK

The providers in this book are listed by state. Each listing includes contact information. I recommend visiting a practitioner's website to read up on what he or she does, and his or her approach to medicine, and then calling the office to ask about insurance and any other questions you might have—that information changes frequently and isn't always up-to-date online. While I have provided the names of the top doctors I found in my own research, it is up to you to select the one you feel comfortable working with and believe will be a great fit for your particular situation.

As you begin (or continue) this journey, you'll find that there are hundreds, if not thousands, of details to keep track of. Staying organized is extremely important, not only because it will reduce your sense of overwhelm, but also because it will help you be as efficient as possible when you do meet with members of your team.

I'd like to offer you one more resource: my Autism Healing Planner video. During the journey to heal your child from autism, as you incorporate the different elements of the Autism Healing Matrix, you'll find that there are tons of pieces of information to keep track of (as you know, the Matrix focuses on diet, a healthcare team, a supportive environment, supplements, educational approaches, probiotics, and celebrating success).

In the Autism Healing Planner video, I show you exactly how to keep track of the details relating to each of the components in the Autism Healing Matrix. This way, when you do get to visit with a Functional Medicine practitioner, your appointments will be as organized and productive as possible! A quick note, here: Your child's healing requires teamwork: a partnership between you, your child's pediatrician, any specialists you work with, and the Functional Medicine practitioner you choose. The best way to play your part successfully is to be organized—to arrive at every appointment with all the necessary information organized and easy to access. (I speak from personal experience here!)

Plus, I'm giving you a checklist of which eight specific organization-related items you need.

Getting and staying organized can be challenging, especially when you're exhausted and stressed. But again, it's really important.

You can watch the video and get the checklist here, at no cost— it's my gift  to you.

TheLyonsReport.com/planner

# IN CLOSING …

**It's my mission and my greatest desire that, as the parent of a child with autism, you feel empowered to help him heal, by taking a compassionate and scientific approach to each step.**

I want you to know that you don't have to stay in the caregiver role. You can step back into the parent role and enjoy parenting again—as your child enjoys his life again!

Remember, healing really *is* possible.

*And you are not alone.*

There are resources available to you that can provide you the information and support you need.

This book is just one of them—to provide you with the names and contact information of Functional Medicine practitioners who want to work with those with autism, and who focus on restoring health and function, not just suppressing symptoms, in the U.S.

I'd love for you to consider *me* a resource, too. I want nothing more than to support as many parents as I can with the expertise I've gained through my own journey with my daughter, and compassion.

I'd like to invite you to learn more about my company, Navigating AWEtism, awetism.net, and to follow my YouTube channel, youtube.awetism.net. I frequently add new videos that contain scientific information as well as inspiration, as I answer questions I receive from parents just like you.

Without further ado, dig in and find a Functional Medicine practitioner who is a good fit for your child … and let the healing begin.

Every step forward matters,

Theresa Lyons MS, MS, PhD

# The Lyons Report: Autism & Functional Medicine Doctors 2020

## ALABAMA

N/A

## ALASKA

N/A

## ARIZONA

**Nic Peters, MD**
2055 East Southern Avenue, Suite H
Tempe, AZ 85282
(480) 704-3446
http://azgoodhealthcenter.com/Team.aspx

**Richard Frye, MD, PhD**
Phoenix Children's Medical Group - Neurology
1919 East Thomas Road
Phoenix, AZ 85016
(602) 933-0970
https://www.phoenixchildrens.org/find-a-doctor/richard-e-frye-md-phd

# ARKANSAS

**N/A**

# CALIFORNIA

**Dan Rossignol, MD**
**Dane Fliedner, MD**
24541 Pacific Park Drive, Suite 210
Aliso Viejo, CA 92656
(321) 259-7111
https://rossignolmedicalcenter.com/

**Richard Chen, MD**
435 Petaluma Avenue, Suite 150
Sebastopol, CA 95472 US
(707) 861-7300
https://hillparkmedicalcenter.com/practitioners/richard/

**Suzanne Goh, MD**
7090 Miratech Drive
San Diego, CA 92121
(858) 304-6440
https://www.corticacare.com

**Lisa Loegering, MD**
327 14th Street
Del Mar, CA 92014
(858) 222-0328
https://www.lisaloegeringmd.com/

**David Traver, MD**
1261 East Hillsdale Blvd, Suite 5
Foster City, CA 94404
(650) 341-5300
http://dptmd.com/

**Donna Ruiz, MD**
29995 Technology Drive, Suite 203
Murrieta, CA 92563
(951) 319-7819 ext 3506
https://donnaruizmd.com/

# COLORADO

**Angie N Martinez, MD**
8670 Wolff Court, Suite 250
Westminster, CO 80031
http://drangiemartinez.com/

# CONNECTICUT

**Nancy O'Hara, MD**
3 Hollyhock Lane
Wilton, CT 06897
(203) 834-2813
http://www.ihealthnow.org/

**Eileen Comia, MD**
35 Jolley Drive, Suite 102
Bloomfield, CT 06002
(860) 264-5188
https://www.advbiomedtx.com/

# DELAWARE

**N/A**

# DISTRICT OF COLUMBIA

**N/A**

# FLORIDA

### Federico J Martinez, MD
3363 NE 163 Street, Suite 809
North Miami Beach, FL 33160
(786) 345-1516
https://www.integrativehealth.us/

### Brian Udell, M.D.
6974 Griffin Road
Davie, FL 33314
(954) 873-8413
http://www.childdev.org/

### Jerry Kartzinel, MD
125 Terra Mango Loop, Suite B
Orlando, FL 32835
(949) 398-7654
https://drjerryk.com/

# GEORGIA

### Juliana Nahas, MD
5211 US Highway 278 NE
Covington, GA 30014
(770) 787-7444
https://www.covingtonpediatrics.com/

**Maia Alees Walton, MD**
1240-A Upper Hembree Road
Roswell, GA 30076
(888) 381-8556
https://www.themwellnesscenter.com/

# HAWAII

**N/A**

# IDAHO

**N/A**

# IOWA

**N/A**

# ILLINOIS

**Peter Kozlowski, MD**
92 Turner Avenue
Elk Grove Village, IL 60007
(847) 626-5758
http://doc-koz.com/

**Anju Usman, MD**
603 East Diehl Road, Suite 135
Naperville, IL 60563
(630) 995-4242
https://www.truehealthmedical.com

# INDIANA

**Mary Lou Hulseman, MD**
9560 East 59th Street
Indianapolis, IN 46216
(317) 621-1700
https://fad.ecommunity.com/provider/

# KANSAS

**Casey Tramp, MD**
8756 151st Street
Overland Park, KS 66221
(913) 380-1903
https://sastundirect.com/

# KENTUCKY

**Anastasia Jandes, MD**
2716 Old Rosebud Road, Suite 230
Lexington, KY 40509
(859) 554-0485
https://theomnihealth.com/

# LOUISIANA

**Joseph Mather, MD**
1504 North Causeway Boulevard
Metairie, LA 70001
(504) 558-4999
http://www.doctormather.com/

**Stephanie Cave, MD**
10562 South Glenstone Place
Baton Rouge, LA 70810
(225) 767-7433
https://stephaniecavemd.com

# MAINE

**N/A**

# MARYLAND

### Phyllis J Heffner, MD
10801 Hickory Ridge Road, Suite 215
Columbia, MD 21044
(410) 260-0344
https://www.holisticchildpsychiatry.com/

# MASSACHUSETTS

### Jeffrey Kreher, MD
255 Low Street, Suite 202
Newburyport, MA 01950
(978) 225-0378
https://www.pcpnewburyport.com/

### Elizabeth Boham, MD
55 Pittsfield Road, Suite 9
Lenox, MA 01240
(413) 637-9991
https://www.ultrawellnesscenter.com

# MICHIGAN

### Mark Leventer, MD
12337 East Michigan Ave.
Grass Lake, MI 49240
(517) 522-8403
https://grasslakemedicalcenter.com/complementary-services/

# MINNESOTA

**Christopher M Foley, MD**
3485 Willow Lake Boulevard, Suite 100
Vadnais Heights, MN 55110
(651) 484-5567
https://minnesotanaturalmedicine.com/

# MISSISSIPPI

N/A

# MISSOURI

N/A

# MONTANA

N/A

# NEBRASKA

N/A

# NEVADA

### Armen Nikogosian, MD
2225 Village Walk Drive #270
Henderson, NV 89052
(702) 616-4001
http://www.autismbiomedcenter.com/

### Scott Jacobson, MD
10120 South Eastern Avenue, Suite 130
Las Vegas, NV 89052
(702) 970-1111
http://www.wishingwellnessmedical.com/

### Amy R Sparks, MD
10155 West Twain, Suite 110
Las Vegas, NV 89147
(702) 722-2200
http://sparksfamilymedicine.com/

# NEW HAMPSHIRE

**N/A**

# NEW JERSEY

**N/A**

# NEW MEXICO

## Carmen Solano, MD
1460 Trinity Drive, Suite 8
Los Alamos, NM 87544
(505) 500-8356
https://infinitywellnessnm.com/

# NEW YORK

## Joseph Malak, MD
207 Washington Street
Poughkeepsie, NY 12601
(845) 249-2510
www.bambini-peds.com/home.html

## Stephen Cowan, MD
26 East 36th Street
New York, NY 10016
(914) 882-9335
http://www.stephencowanmd.com/

## Michael E. Gabriel, MD
8120 15th Avenue
Brooklyn, NY 11209
(718) 256-2555
https://gpmpediatrics.com/Home

**Raphael Kellman, MD**
7 West 45th Street, Suite 301
New York, NY 10036
(212) 717-1118
https://kellmancenter.com/

# NORTH CAROLINA

**Diana Roberson, MD**
425 South Sharon Amity Road , Suite B
Charlotte, NC 28211
(980) 260-0900
https://livingwaterpediatrics.com

**Novlet Davis, MD**
875 Walnut Street, Suite 275-9
Cary, NC 27540
(919) 749-6288
http://www.autismtreatmentcenterofraleigh.com/

**Karen Harum, MD**
5725 Oleander Drive, SuiteC-1
Wilmington, NC 28403
(910) 319-7744
http://www.clinicforspecialchildren.net/

**Anne Hines, MD**
3000 Bethesda Place
Winston-Salem, NC 27103
(336) 896-0954
https://www.annehinesmd.com/

# NORTH DAKOTA

N/A

# OHIO

**Anup Kanodia, MD**
5003 Pine Creek Drive
Columbus, OH 43081 US
(614) 524-4527
https://kanodiamd.com/

**Deborah Nash, MD**
245 South Garber Drive
Tipp City, OH 45371
(937) 877-1222
http://www.nashintegrativemedicine.com/

# OKLAHOMA

**N/A**

# OREGON

**John Green, MD**
516 High Street
Oregon City, OR 97045
(503) 722-4270
https://childrenandautism.com/

# PENNSYLVANIA

**Nadia Ali, MD**
993 Old Eagle School Road, Suite 311
West Chester, PA 19380
(267)250-3676
https://www.theholistichealing.org/autism

**Simona Manuela Walsh, MD**
253 West State Street, Suite B
Doylestown, PA 18901
(267) 454-7262
http://www.bcimedicine.com/

# RHODE ISLAND

**N/A**

# SOUTH CAROLINA

**N/A**

# SOUTH DAKOTA

**N/A**

# TENNESSEE

**Eric Potter, MD**
120 Holiday Court, Suite 2
Franklin, TN 37067
(615) 721-2001
https://sanctuaryfunctionalmedicine.com/

# TEXAS

**Paula Kruppstadt, MD**
150 Pine Forest Drive, Suite 701
Shenandoah, TX 77384
(281) 725-6767
https://get2theroot.com/

**Elizabeth Suarez, MD**
3201 University Drive East, Suite 425
Bryan, TX 77802
(979) 690-4828
https://www.chistjoseph.org/

**Randy Naidoo, MD**
**Rahima Afroza, MD**
3600 Shire Boulevard, Suite 110
Richardson, Texas 75082
(469) 333-1543
https://www.shinepediatrics.com

**Deborah Z. Bain, MD**
4851 Legacy Drive, Suite #301
Frisco, Texas 75034
(972) 294-0808
http://www.healthykidspediatrics.com/

**Alina Olteanu, MD**
3550 Parkwood Blvd, Suite 100
Frisco, Texas 75034
(214) 736-1954
http://www.wholechildtexas.com/

**Anand Dilip Bhatt, MD**
400 West Lyndon B Johnson Freeway, Plaza I, Suite 250
Irving, TX 75063
(972) 481-6400
https://www.bswhealth.com/physician/anand-bhatt

# UTAH

**Drew Christensen, MD**
1755 Prospector Avenue, Suite 100
Park City, UT 84060
(435) 214-7282
https://heartofyourhealth.com/

# VERMONT

**N/A**

# VIRGINIA

**April Guminsky, MD**
121 Bulifants Boulevard, Suite A
Williamsburg, VA 23188
(757) 707-3025
http://www.gatewaymedpeds.com/

**Elizabeth Mumper, MD**
2919 Confederate Ave.
Lynchburg, VA 24501
(434) 528-9075
https://www.rimlandcenter.com/

**Eric Madren, MD**
725 Volvo Parkway, Suite 100
Chesapeake, VA 23320
(757) 548-0076
https://www.bayviewphysicians.com/physician/eric-madren/

**Eric Rydland, MD**
1524 Insurance Lane
Charlottesville, VA 22911
(434) 984-5437
https://rydlandpediatrics.com/

**Mary Megson, MD**
7229 Forest Avenue, Suite 211
Richmond, VA 23226
(804) 673-9128
http://www.megson.com/

**Margaret Gennaro, MD**
10560 Main Street, Suite 301
Fairfax, VA 22030
(703) 865-5692
http://www.drmgennaro.com/

# WASHINGTON

### Monica German, MD
922 South Cowley Street, Suite 7
Spokane, WA 99202
(509) 262-8145
http://medicine-naturally.com/

### Carol Doroshow, M.D.
4411 Fremont Avenue North
Seattle, WA 98103
(206) 957-1881
https://www.thekidsclinic.us/

### Megan Debell, MD
1633 Bellevue Avenue, Suite A
Seattle, WA 98122
(206) 734-8370
https://www.shinefunctionalmedicine.com/about.html

# WEST VIRGINIA

**N/A**

# WISCONSIN

**Aruna K. Tummala, MD**
12800 West National Avenue
New Berlin, WI 53151
(262) 955-6601
https://trinergyhealth.com/

# WYOMING

**N/A**

Made in USA - Crawfordsville, IN
12545_9781734358209
03.18.2020 1548